Find Your Inner Ninja

Learning to Embrace Your Life's Journey

Parisjat Umscheid

<u>Dedication</u>

For my husband, Steve - this journey called life
would not be half as fun or exciting if you were
not with me

For my three kids - Karenna, Lucy and Brody -
you are my Ninja Inspiration - I love you more
than I could ever express in life

For Cindy - you are missed my Crossfit twin

Introduction

My name is Parisjat and I am from Thailand. I married my American husband 14 years ago and am now a 44 year old suburban mom of three kids. I was born in Paris and my grandfather was the former Prime Minister of Thailand, Pridi Banomyong. Somehow I feel like this is exactly how my life is supposed to be.

I grew up in the most traditional Asian families. If you know about the book called *"Hymn of the Tiger Mom"* that caused a lot of controversy when it came out. Then you know a little bit about what it means to be born in a traditional Asian family. In fact when I read it, I actually thought this was my mom writing this book.

I grew up with very strict mother who had high expectations of me to be this perfect daughter who excelled in academics. And, of course, I was not the perfect daughter because I was not very gifted in the academic world but I was showed a talent in sports. So much to her dismay she really didn't know what to do with me when I started doing sports in high school. As you can imagine that was a big struggle between us. It still continues to this day.

Growing up in a traditional Asian household and being expected to do well in school I felt like I was a rebel or the black sheep of the family because I went towards sports. Now I was lucky enough that my dad was very encouraging with me. He was a kind of buffer between my mom and I and our relationship.

Fast-forward I came to America for school and went to college. In college I didn't really continue my sporting journey. I fell into the whole American lifestyle. For me it was the freshmen fifty not freshman 15. I didn't actually get back into fitness until after the birth of my third child at the age of 35

The fitness gap in my life is pretty understandable and to

many relatable. After getting married I had three kids within four years.   As you can be imagine that can take a toll on a women's life. After the weight that I had gained from the birth of my third child, I knew I had to do something about it. As I looked back at my life I began to realize that the person I had always been was somebody who really had embraced and loved fitness and athletics. What happened to her I would wonder as I sat on the couch late at night with my glass of wine and double scoop of ice-cream.

Setting a BIG Goal

I decided that I was going to get off the couch and I was going to do whatever it took to get back into shape. I just decided that I would start running. The first few weeks were really tough! I didn't really run, I just walked. And then slowly I started to run.

I decided that in order for me to accomplish my goals I had to set a goal that was so big that it almost seemed impossible, at first. So I set a goal to do a marathon before my son turned one. I would do whatever it took to get out and run . Sometimes early in the morning before everybody woke up or late at night when everyone was asleep. I knew that with training for a marathon, there are no shortcuts. You have to sign up for a marathon and show up on the day and think and hope that all your training will pay off and that you are ready. This worked for me. There was a progression and there was a plan. For my personality that seemed to work. I really need a weekly plan to hold me accountable. A step by step guide on how to complete a marathon.

I'm very happy to say that I did do my first marathon when my son was almost exactly a year. After that I really realized that sweating and working out became my stress reliever. Exercise was an instant release from the demands of being a stay at home mom. With three kids under the age of 4,I was knee deep in diaper duty and sleepless nights.

After the marathon, I decided I like to challenge myself again. I decided to dabble in triathlons. So once again I had a plan. I knew I needed a way to track my progress. When I met my triathlon training goals, I looked for the next thing I could do to challenge myself. I discovered CrossFit. For those who aren't familiar with CrossFit, it is known for high intensity and challenging workouts. With Crossfit you could not specialize in one thing, you had to train all your weakness and strength within one workout. For some reason CrossFit came into my life at the right time because it changed my life, my family's life and it is the reason that I am the person I am today.

Cindy- Don't Wait

The key in each of these was to take it one step at a time and get me from where I was, to a person who could do a marathon or someone who could do triathlons or Crossfit. I found a new sense of purpose and a greater sense of me being myself. Crossfit literally made me a better person. It taught me to embrace my strength and be proud of who I had become. It also was where I met a beautiful lady named Cindy.

Cindy and I used to joke that we are Crossfit Twins. We had so much in common. We were both moms of three kids. We both were Asian and we are both vertically challenged. Most importantly, we both love CrossFit.

Cindy went to a different Crossfit location then I did and I would always see her at local Crossfit competitions for the past 5 years.

By this time I had decided to obtain my Crossfit Level 1 Certification so that I could be a CrossFit coach. The reason was that I really wanted to bring CrossFit to the schools and have kids be moving in an after-school fun fitness program. That is really important to me -to get kids more active.

Our Crossfit community found out about Cindy's illness when

she announced on her Facebook page in January of 2015 that she had been diagnosed with stage-4 lung cancer. Someone so young, beautiful healthy and fit was sick. I cannot express how deeply her passing affected those who knew her. She touched and inspired by her smile, her love of her family and the Crossfit community she was a part of. Sadly, she just passed away on September 3rd 2015. She was so full of life. She was an amazing athlete.

Cindy had a message that she gave all of us. Her simple message was, "Live your life fully and don't wait." Cindy's words I carry with me in my wallet. It is a constant encouragement and reminder to me to live my life fully each day and to not wait!

The Next American Ninja Warrior

Now our family loves watching the hit NBC Show 'The Next American Ninja Warrior.' It's something fun for us to all watch together. In the afterschool fitness class I teach to kids in elementary school, my students are always coming up to me saying, "Coach P, I think you should be the next American Ninja Warrior." I would always laugh it off and say, "Coach P is way too old to be an American Ninja Warrior.

This is where our excuses come in, because at age 44 and soon to be considered middle age, I was telling myself that American Ninja Warrior is for the young kids. But when Cindy passed away, I really thought about her message of living life fully and not waiting. I thought, "Why am I waiting? I need to train to be the next American Ninja Warrior. There is no reason why I shouldn't do it." If there is a plan and trackable progression, then I know that I can do it. I've proven that I can achieve my fitness goals with a plan and progression.

So right now that has become my new journey and my reason to wake up and work on my dreams, I want to be the next American Ninja Warrior.

Really what my journey is all about is living your life as fully as you can. For me I tend to base my decision so that when I'm 70 or 80 and I look back on my life I can say yes to the question, "Did I do everything I could do at the time?" For me, age is really just a number because my body still allows me to move and to move pretty well. I don't want to look back when I'm 80 and say, "Why didn't I try to do this when my body would let me?"

I don't know if at 80 I'm going to be able to get up and do pull ups and go rock climbing. However, in my 40s, I still have a good shot. I made my decisions so I can look back on my life and have no regret.

Even in the days when it seems daunting and challenging, as long as I can see that I am making progress and improvement on then I keep going and I keep showing up.

I focus on the progress. I take each thing step by step. This is the only way to keep going. You focus on the challenge for today and what you are able to do in the moment.

Sharing Your Journey

My hope is that what I am doing is inspiring and motivating others to dream big. If I can motivate even one person then all of this would be worth it. I am so blessed to be surrounded with a supportive community of people. They keep me motivated to not give up, not matter how hard.

Cindy's message was to live your life fully every day. I wake up and do that every day. The way that I am going to reach my big dream isn't by waking up tomorrow and jumping on the course and succeeding from day one. We have to have a step by step plan. These step by step plans are what helps people get from where they are to where they want to go.

After my first seventy five days now of having been training to being a Ninja Warrior, what I've learned is that you have to tell everyone what your goal is. You've got to share it with the world so that the world holds you accountable to it, but also so that people in your life have the opportunity to be able to help. The truth is if we tell nobody, it would be so easy to walk away when things got too difficult or you find that you really don't have the time. This doesn't have to apply only to becoming an American Ninja Warrior, this could be for anything that you want to do to make your life better.

You want to invite people into your life. You want to share your goals with them. Share with your support community each next step. When you tell your supporters, "Tomorrow I am going to do X." They will then hold you accountable. They will become a part of your journey. They become part of your motivation.The support from others helps you not only succeed but it helps them be encouraged by your journey.

You'll find that other people do want you to succeed. They want to find out what they can do to help. They want to be there to watch you, to support you, to encourage you and to see you succeed.

This applies whether you want to do your first 5K or you've decided that you also want to start down the journey of being the next American Ninja Warrior. There will be people at the same level on your journey that you are. These people would love to connect with you and do it alongside of you as you take your journey. They will check in on you and they will ask you. How is your training going? Or are you getting to your next goal? And it makes you feel that you have someone to answer to.

When you do have something you want to accomplish, I feel that you need to shout it to the world. Tell everyone that you meet, even if someone gives you a weird look. I've had that. I had people look at me and say, "Really? Is this for real?" Yes, it is for real. If you don't tell anyone it's so easy to give up because nobody knew about it. But if you tell people and you share with people it creates an accountability factor. You will find that you want to do well, not just for yourself but for people who support. To me I found that to be very important. Don't be shy about what you want, let everybody know.

Involving My Kids

Now here is the thing, I'm still a mom, I'm still a wife. My children are in grade school and middle school, so I still have my responsibilities. What I've had to do is find ways that I can get my family involved. The kids help me scope out playgrounds. I take parkour and gymnastic classes with them .My kids will say, "Mom, have you tried this?" And they'll do some stuff that I've never seen done before on the monkey bars. Involving my kids in this journey makes it not only fun but creating memories as a family.

One thing I can guarantee you is that your kids will hold you accountable. Whether it be in a fitness journey or a weight loss journey or something new you want to try. If you tell your kids, I can guarantee you that they are going to come back to you and ask you how you are doing. They will hold you accountable to the commitment that you've made. My kids love commenting on what food they think is ninja approved or not ninja approved. It is a lot of fun to say, "Mom, are you sure you should be having that ice cream? Is that ninja approved?"

What I've found in my journey is that this is a way that I can play with my kids every day. I just literally incorporate the journey that I'm on into my ability to be able to spend time with my kids in a fun way. And on the days when I don't feel like it, they are more than happy to nag me into getting out there and getting it done.

Embrace the Journey

What I've learned is that you have to embrace the journey, not the results. You have to set your mind on the current experience and not just the outcome. Be patient with the process. It's not going to happen immediately. You are not going to wake up tomorrow and be at your goal. But each step, each day, you can get a little bit closer. This is where I am now, this is where I was and this is where I'm going. Each day just needs to help you get one step closer to your big dream.

I want to be able to say I'm going to be a Ninja Warrior and

I want to be able to run up that wall immediately. Well that isn't going to happen unless I put in the work to get there. So what I've learned now is to really just embrace where I'm at now because this is my starting point and every day is a chance to get better.

Keep in mind that there are the good days and bad days. There are some days that it's just hard and not fun. But if you emphasize in your mind the good days and celebrate the little victories. It can help you get through the tough times. When your day and training is not going well - and it happens - think of something you accomplished and hold onto that image in your mind.

Handling Life's Challenges

We all have time challenges. As a stay at home mom and also starting up a company and being a wife, I understand that there are things that take up our time. Things will come up to keep you from reaching your goal.

Don't let the challenges in your life keep you from being the best YOU that YOU can be. I want you to understand that it's important for you to make yourself a priority. It is okay to take time away from your family. It's okay to make time for your goals in your life as well. You don't need to be lost in the duties of being a wife and a mom. All of us as moms put our kids first and we often fall into the trap of not doing anything for ourselves. But I want you to know that you can take time for you. It's okay to have ME time. If you will embrace that, you then can begin an exciting new journey.

We need to embrace the power of our mind. Our mind can actually be our most powerful ally or our biggest enemy. If you believe in yourself, you can achieve things. But you have to believe in yourself. If you don't believe in yourself, your mind will tell you all the reasons why you can't do it. If you do believe in yourself, your mind can help you through things that your body doesn't feel like it can even do. Because your mind is so much more powerful than your body.

What we need to learn to do is to program our minds. We need to learn what to say to ourselves to make ourselves go that next step on our journey. Then your mind will tell your body what to do.

Don't forget who you are and what your dreams are. Because you need to be the hero in your own story. You need to embrace that your journey may be the answer to someone else's prayers. You never know who is watching and who will be inspired by you.

Step by Step

So here is what you need to do. Today I want to encourage you to be the best version of yourself. Start off by making a list. What did you like to do as a child? There may be a big gap like there was in my life of not doing what I used to love, but that is okay. You can still embrace what you love to do at any age. You can find your true passion by finding those things that as a child you used to love to do. Then you can find ways to put it into the context of your current life.

We have to start with baby steps, but you have to take action. Ask yourself, "What can I do today?" Because I believe that anyone can accomplish anything at any age, they just have to begin to start.

So first we are going to decide what it is that we are passionate about. Then we are going to set a goal for ourselves. Then we are going to start telling everybody. We want to involve others. We want to surround ourselves with supporters and try to make everyone we come in contact with a part of our tribe. Give your followers ways that they can engage with you, because you can't do it alone.

The key to success is community. It takes a village

to make a ninja. It's not a secret, it's a declaration.

You Can Do It!

Embrace the journey in your life. Follow what is in your heart.

It's not about what is expected of you. It's not about the traditions of your family. It's not about what your mom or dad thought you should be. It's not about what everybody like you is supposed to be. It's about being the best version of you.

You are not training, you are not taking on your next goal for your mom. You are doing it for you. Keep in mind that it's not about the end result, it's about being present in the moment.

As my friend Cindy said, "Live your life fully." One of my favorite workout shirts I workout in says, "I can. I will." Four words. I encourage you today to embrace.

Take the challenge in your life today to accept the challenge of a new goal. Accept a new journey that you can to take right now in your life. Then say to yourself, "I can. I will. Forward."

I believe in you!
You can do it!
I'll be watching and cheering for you!